CANCER DIET SOLUTION:

Nourish Your Body, Fight Disease

Aveah J Smith

Table of Contents

Introduction

Welcome to "The Cancer Diet Solution: Nourish Your Body, Fight Disease." In this book, we will explore the powerful connection between nutrition and cancer, and how you can use food as a tool to support your body's fight against this disease.

Cancer is a complex and challenging condition that affects millions of lives worldwide. While medical treatments play a crucial role in cancer care, the impact of nutrition on prevention, treatment, and recovery should not be underestimated. Research has shown that certain dietary choices can influence cancer risk, support the body's immune system, and enhance overall well-being during and after treatment.

In this book, we will delve into the science behind the relationship between nutrition and cancer. We will explore the key nutrients, superfoods, and dietary components that have been shown to have cancer-fighting properties. You will learn how to build a cancer-fighting plate, incorporating a variety of wholesome foods that nourish your body and provide the necessary nutrients for optimal health.

Meal planning is an essential aspect of a cancer-fighting diet, and we will guide you through the process of creating balanced and nutritious meal plans. We will provide sample meal plans, recipe ideas, and practical tips to help you incorporate these dietary changes into your daily life.

It is important to note that this book is not a substitute for medical advice or treatment. We encourage you to work closely with your healthcare team, including oncologists, nutritionists, and dietitians, to develop a personalized approach that suits your specific needs and treatment plan.

By embracing a cancer-fighting lifestyle through food, you have the power to make positive changes in your life. Through nourishing your body with wholesome ingredients, practicing mindful eating, and prioritizing self-care, you can support your overall health and well-being during and beyond cancer treatment.

Let's embark on this journey together and discover how the right nutrition can nourish your body and help you fight disease.

Chapter 1

Understanding Cancer and Nutrition

In this chapter, we will delve into the intricate relationship between cancer and nutrition. By understanding how nutrition impacts cancer development, progression, and treatment outcomes, we can make informed choices to support our health and well-being. Some of the topics covered in this chapter include:

The Link Between Nutrition and Cancer: We will explore the scientific evidence that highlights the connection between nutrition and cancer. This includes the role of certain dietary factors in promoting or inhibiting cancer growth.

Lifestyle Factors and Cancer Risk: Discussing the impact of lifestyle factors, such as diet, physical activity, smoking, and alcohol consumption, on cancer risk. We will examine how making positive changes in these areas can reduce the risk of developing certain types of cancer.

Key Nutrients for Cancer Prevention and Treatment: Highlighting the importance of specific nutrients in supporting the body's defense against cancer. We will discuss the role of antioxidants, vitamins, minerals, fiber, and phytochemicals in promoting cellular health and reducing cancer risk. The Influence of Diet on Cancer Treatment: Exploring how nutrition can impact the effectiveness of cancer treatments, such as chemotherapy, radiation therapy, and immunotherapy. We will discuss the importance of maintaining adequate nutrition during treatment to support the body's ability to heal and recover. Addressing Common Nutritional Challenges: Discussing common dietary challenges faced by cancer patients, such as loss of appetite, taste changes, and digestive issues. We will provide strategies and tips to overcome these challenges and ensure adequate nutrition during treatment. Integrative Approaches: Exploring the integration of nutrition with conventional cancer treatments and complementary therapies. We will discuss how nutrition can be used as a complementary approach to enhance treatment outcomes and improve overall well-being.

The Role of Medical Professionals and Nutritionists: Highlighting the importance of collaboration between healthcare providers and nutrition experts in developing personalized dietary plans for cancer patients. We will discuss the role of oncologists, nutritionists, and dietitians in providing guidance and support throughout the cancer journey.

Empowering Patients and Caregivers: Encouraging active participation in dietary decision-making and providing resources for informed food choices. We will discuss the importance of self-advocacy and the role of caregivers in supporting the nutritional needs of cancer patients. It is important to note that while nutrition plays a significant role in cancer prevention and treatment, it is not a standalone solution. It should be integrated with medical treatments and personalized care plans. By understanding the relationship between cancer and nutrition, we can make informed choices to support our health and well-being throughout the cancer journey.

Chapter 2

Building a Cancer-Fighting Plate

In this chapter, we will explore the principles of building a cancer-fighting plate. By incorporating a variety of nutrient-dense foods into our meals, we can support our body's defense against cancer and promote overall health. Some of the topics covered in this chapter include:

Principles of a Cancer-Fighting Diet: We will discuss the key principles of a cancer-fighting diet, which include focusing on whole foods, incorporating a variety of fruits and vegetables, choosing lean proteins, opting for healthy fats, and selecting whole grains.

Portion Sizes and Macronutrient Balance: Understanding portion sizes and balancing macronutrients (carbohydrates, proteins, and fats) is essential for maintaining a healthy diet. We will provide guidance on portion control and tips for achieving a balanced plate.

Incorporating Fruits and Vegetables: Fruits and vegetables are rich in vitamins, minerals, antioxidants, and fiber, making them essential components of a cancer-fighting plate. We will discuss the importance of incorporating a variety of colorful fruits and vegetables into our meals and provide tips on how to increase their consumption.

Choosing Lean Proteins: Protein is crucial for cell repair and growth, and choosing lean sources of protein is important for a cancer-fighting diet. We will explore options such as poultry, fish, legumes, and plant-based proteins, and discuss their benefits.

Opting for Healthy Fats: Healthy fats, such as those found in avocados, nuts, seeds, and olive oil, provide essential nutrients and support overall health. We will discuss the importance of incorporating these fats into our diet and provide tips on how to do so.

Selecting Whole Grains: Whole grains are rich in fiber, vitamins, minerals, and antioxidants. We will discuss the benefits of choosing whole grains over refined grains and provide examples of whole grain options to include in our meals.

Hydration and Cancer Prevention: Staying hydrated is crucial for overall health and can help reduce the risk of certain cancers. We will discuss the importance of hydration, provide tips on how to increase water intake, and explore other hydrating options.

Mindful Eating: Mindful eating involves paying attention to our body's hunger and fullness cues, as well as savoring and enjoying our meals. We will discuss the benefits of mindful eating and provide tips on how to incorporate it into our daily routine.

By building a cancer-fighting plate, we can

nourish our bodies with the essential nutrients

needed to support our health and well-being.

Through a balanced and varied diet, we can

optimize our body's ability to fight against

cancer and promote overall wellness.

Chapter 3

Superfoods for Cancer Prevention and Healing

In this chapter, we will explore the concept of superfoods and their potential role in cancer prevention and healing. Superfoods are nutrient-dense foods that are rich in antioxidants, vitamins, minerals, and other beneficial compounds. Including these foods in our diet can provide additional support for our body's defense against cancer. Some of the topics covered in this chapter include:

Introduction to Superfoods: We will define what superfoods are and discuss their potential benefits for cancer prevention and healing. We will emphasize the importance of incorporating a variety of superfoods into our diet to maximize their health benefits.

Berries: Nature's Antioxidant Powerhouses:

Berries, such as blueberries, strawberries, raspberries, and blackberries, are packed with antioxidants that can help protect our cells from damage and reduce inflammation. We will explore the specific health benefits of different types of berries and provide ideas on how to incorporate them into our meals and snacks.

Cruciferous Vegetables: A Crucial Defense Against Cancer: Cruciferous vegetables, including broccoli, cauliflower, kale, Brussels sprouts, and cabbage, contain compounds that have been shown to have anti-cancer properties. We will discuss the potential benefits of these vegetables and provide recipes and cooking tips to help you incorporate them into your diet.

Turmeric: The Golden Spice for Fighting Inflammation: Turmeric contains a compound called curcumin, which has powerful anti-inflammatory and antioxidant properties. We will explore the potential benefits of turmeric in cancer prevention and healing and provide ideas on how to include it in your meals.

Green Tea: A Sip of Health and Protection: Green tea is rich in antioxidants called catechins, which have been associated with a reduced risk of certain types of cancer. We will discuss the potential benefits of green tea and provide tips on how to incorporate it into your daily routine.

Other Superfoods for Cancer Prevention and Healing: In addition to berries, cruciferous vegetables, turmeric, and green tea, there are many other superfoods that can support our body's defense against cancer. We will explore foods such as garlic, mushrooms, leafy greens, nuts, seeds, and more, and discuss their potential benefits.

By incorporating superfoods into our diet, we can provide our bodies with an extra boost of nutrients and compounds that support our overall health and well-being. While superfoods are not a cure for cancer, they can be a valuable addition to a balanced and varied diet that promotes cancer prevention and healing.

Chapter 4

Meal Planning for Cancer-Fighting Success

In this chapter, we will dive into the importance of meal planning for a cancer-fighting diet. Meal planning is a valuable tool that can help ensure you have nutritious and balanced meals throughout the week, even during busy times. We will provide practical tips, ... strategies, and sample meal plans to support your journey towards optimal health. Some of the topics covered in this chapter include:

The Importance of Meal Planning: We will discuss the benefits of meal planning, including saving time, reducing stress, and promoting healthier food choices. By planning your meals in advance, you can ensure that you have the necessary ingredients on hand and ... avoid relying on unhealthy convenience foods.

Creating Balanced and Nutritious Meal Plans: We will guide you through the process of creating balanced and nutritious meal plans that support your cancer-fighting goals. We will discuss the importance of incorporating a variety of food groups, such as fruits, vegetables, whole grains, ... lean proteins, and healthy fats, into your meals.

Sample Meal Plans for Different Stages of Cancer Treatment: We will provide sample meal plans tailored to different stages of cancer treatment, such as pre-treatment, during treatment, and post-treatment. These meal plans will take into account the specific nutritional needs and challenges that may arise ... during each stage. We will provide ideas for breakfast, lunch, dinner, and snacks, ensuring that you have a variety of options to choose from.

Grocery Shopping Guide for Cancer-Fighting Ingredients: We will provide guidance on navigating the grocery store and selecting cancer-fighting ingredients. We will discuss the importance of reading food labels, choosing fresh produce, selecting healthy proteins, and stocking up on pantry staples. ... We will also provide tips on meal prepping and batch cooking to make your meal planning process more efficient.

Adapting Meal Plans for Dietary Preferences and Restrictions: We understand that everyone has unique dietary preferences and restrictions. We will provide guidance on how to adapt the sample meal plans to accommodate different dietary needs, such as vegetarian, vegan, gluten-free, or dairy-free.

... We will also discuss ingredient substitutions for common allergens or dietary restrictions, ensuring that you can still enjoy delicious and nutritious meals.

By incorporating meal planning into your cancer-fighting lifestyle, you can take control of your nutrition and ensure that you are nourishing your body with the right foods. With the guidance and strategies provided in this chapter, you will be equipped to create personalized meal plans that support your health and well-being throughout your cancer journey.

Chapter 5

Cooking Techniques for Maximum Nutrient Retention

In this chapter, we will explore cooking techniques that help preserve the nutritional value of foods, ensuring that you get the most out of your meals. Some of the topics covered in this chapter include:

Steaming: Steaming is a gentle cooking method that helps retain the nutrients in vegetables, fish, and poultry. We will discuss the benefits of steaming and provide tips on how to steam foods properly.

Stir-Frying: Stir-frying is a quick cooking method that uses high heat and minimal oil. This technique helps retain the nutrients in vegetables while adding flavor and texture. We will discuss the best practices for stir-frying and provide recipe ideas.

Roasting: Roasting is a dry heat cooking method that brings out the natural flavors of vegetables and meats. We will discuss how to roast foods to retain their nutrients and provide tips on seasoning and flavoring.

Blanching: Blanching involves briefly boiling vegetables and then plunging them into ice water to stop the cooking process. This technique helps preserve the color, texture, and nutrients of vegetables. We will discuss the blanching process and its benefits.

Raw Preparation: Raw foods can be a great way to maximize nutrient intake. We will discuss the benefits of raw foods, provide tips on safely consuming raw foods, and share recipe ideas for raw dishes.

Using Minimal Water: Cooking foods in minimal water helps retain their nutrients. We will discuss techniques such as sautéing, braising, and using a minimal amount of water for boiling.

Proper Storage and Reheating: Proper storage and reheating techniques can help preserve the nutrients in cooked foods. We will provide tips on storing leftovers and reheating them to maintain their nutritional value.

By incorporating these cooking techniques into your meal preparation, you can ensure that you are maximizing the nutrient retention in your foods and supporting your overall health and well-being during your cancer-fighting journey.

Chapter 6

Mindful Eating for Optimal Health

In this chapter, we will explore the concept of mindful eating and its impact on our overall health and well-being. Mindful eating involves paying attention to our food choices, eating habits, and body's signals. By practicing mindful eating, we can develop a healthier relationship with food, make conscious choices, and fully enjoy the eating experience. Some of the topics covered in this chapter include:

The Power of Mindful Eating: We will discuss the benefits of mindful eating, including improved digestion, better portion control, and increased satisfaction with meals. We will explore how mindful eating can help us reconnect with our body's hunger and fullness cues and promote a more balanced approach to eating.

Strategies for Practicing Mindful Eating: We will provide practical strategies and techniques for incorporating mindful eating into our daily lives. This may include slowing down while eating, savoring each bite, and paying attention to the sensory experience of food. We will also discuss the importance of creating a calm and ... environment for meals and reducing distractions while eating.

Listening to Your Body's Hunger and Fullness Cues: Understanding our body's signals of hunger and fullness is essential for mindful eating. We will explore how to tune in to these cues and eat in response to our body's needs, rather than external factors like emotions or external cues.

Overcoming Emotional Eating: Emotional eating can be a challenge for many individuals. We will discuss strategies for identifying emotional triggers, finding alternative coping mechanisms, and developing a healthier relationship with food.

Mindful Eating and Weight Management:
Mindful eating can be a helpful tool for weight management. We will discuss how mindful eating can support a balanced approach to weight management, focusing on nourishing our bodies and ... rather than restrictive diets or quick fixes.

By practicing mindful eating, we can cultivate a healthier and more enjoyable relationship with food. This chapter will provide you with the knowledge and tools to incorporate mindful eating into your daily life, promoting optimal health and well-being.

Chapter 7

Exercise and Lifestyle Factors for Cancer Prevention

In this chapter, we will explore the importance of exercise and other lifestyle factors in cancer prevention. While nutrition plays a significant role in reducing cancer risk, incorporating regular physical activity and adopting a healthy lifestyle can further enhance our overall well-being and ... reduce the likelihood of developing certain types of cancer. Some of the topics covered in this chapter include:

The Role of Exercise in Cancer Prevention: We will discuss the numerous benefits of exercise in reducing the risk of cancer. Regular physical activity can help maintain a healthy weight, improve immune function, reduce inflammation, and regulate hormone levels. We will explore the ... types of exercise that are most beneficial for cancer prevention and provide practical tips on how to incorporate exercise into your daily routine.

Stress Management and its Impact on Cancer Risk: Chronic stress can have a negative impact on our health, including increasing the risk of cancer. We will discuss the connection between stress and cancer and provide strategies for managing stress effectively. This may include ... techniques such as meditation, deep breathing exercises, yoga, or engaging in hobbies and activities that promote relaxation.

Quality Sleep and its Connection to Overall Well-being: Adequate sleep is essential for our overall health and well-being, including cancer prevention. We will discuss the importance of quality sleep in maintaining a healthy immune system, regulating hormone levels, and supporting cellular repair. We ... will provide tips for improving sleep hygiene and establishing a bedtime routine that promotes restful sleep.

Other Lifestyle Factors for Cancer Prevention: In addition to exercise, stress management, and sleep, we will explore other lifestyle factors that can contribute to cancer prevention. This may include maintaining a healthy weight, avoiding tobacco and excessive alcohol consumption, and protecting ... yourself from excessive sun exposure. We will provide practical tips and strategies for incorporating these lifestyle factors into your daily life.

By incorporating regular exercise and adopting a healthy lifestyle, you can further reduce your risk of developing cancer and promote overall well-being. This chapter will provide you with the knowledge and tools to make positive lifestyle changes that support your cancer prevention efforts.

Chapter 8

Supportive Therapies and Resources

In this chapter, we will explore various supportive therapies and resources that can complement traditional cancer treatments and enhance overall well-being. Some of the topics covered in this chapter include:

Complementary Therapies: We will discuss different complementary therapies such as acupuncture, massage therapy, yoga, and meditation.

These therapies can help manage symptoms, reduce stress, and improve quality of life during cancer treatment.

Support Groups and Counseling: We will explore the benefits of joining support groups and seeking counseling services. These resources provide emotional support, a sense of community, and a safe space to express feelings and concerns.

Integrative Medicine: We will delve into the field of integrative medicine, which combines conventional medical treatments with evidence-based complementary therapies. We will discuss the potential benefits of integrative medicine in cancer care and provide information on finding qualified practitioners.

Online Resources and Apps: We will highlight reputable online resources and mobile applications that offer information, support, and tools for cancer patients and their caregivers.

These resources can provide valuable information, connect you with others going through similar experiences, and offer practical tools for managing your health. By exploring these supportive therapies and resources, you can enhance your cancer treatment journey, improve your well-being, and find additional support during this challenging time.

Conclusion

Embracing a Cancer-Fighting Lifestyle

In this book, we have explored the power of nutrition and lifestyle choices in supporting a cancer-fighting lifestyle. By understanding the link between nutrition and cancer, we can make informed choices to nourish our bodies and promote overall well-being.

We have discussed the importance of building a cancer-fighting plate, incorporating superfoods, meal planning, and embracing a variety of cooking methods to maximize the nutritional value of our meals.

Additionally, we have highlighted the significance of exercise, stress management, sleep, and other lifestyle factors in cancer prevention and overall health. By incorporating regular physical activity, managing stress, prioritizing quality sleep, and making positive lifestyle changes, we can further reduce our risk of developing cancer and support our body's natural defense mechanisms.

Throughout this book, we have emphasized the importance of personalized approaches and working closely with healthcare professionals to develop a comprehensive cancer-fighting plan. It is crucial to consult with oncologists, nutritionists, and other experts to tailor dietary and lifestyle recommendations to your specific needs and treatment plan.

Remember, embracing a cancer-fighting lifestyle is not a one-time effort but a lifelong commitment. It requires dedication, perseverance, and a willingness to make positive changes. By nourishing our bodies with wholesome foods, engaging in regular physical activity, managing stress, prioritizing sleep, and seeking support, we can empower ourselves to take an active role in our health and well-being.

While this book provides valuable information and guidance, it is essential to remember that it is not a substitute for medical advice or treatment. Always consult with your healthcare team for personalized recommendations and support.

By embracing a cancer-fighting lifestyle, we have the power to make positive changes in our lives. Through nourishing our bodies, engaging in regular physical activity, managing stress, prioritizing sleep, and seeking support, we can support our overall health and well-being during and beyond cancer treatment. Every small step towards a healthier lifestyle is a step towards a brighter future.

Let us embark on this journey together and embrace a cancer-fighting lifestyle that promotes optimal health and well-being.